INGROWN TOENAIL

EXPLORING ALL THE ALTERNATIVE FOR
TREATING INGROWN TOENAIL

DR. A. RAMOS

1

Contents

INTRODUCTION

A frequent ailment known as an ingrown toenail occurs when a toenail's edge or corner grows into the surrounding skin. This can lead to pain, irritation, and occasionally infection. Though it can affect any toe, the big toe is the most frequently affected. Ingrown toenails can cause discomfort and, if left untreated, can develop difficulties.

An ingrown toenail frequently results from the nail curving and penetrating the surrounding skin, causing discomfort and swelling. An injury to the toe, tight shoes, incorrect nail cutting, or a genetic tendency can all lead to the formation of ingrown toenails.

An ingrown toenail frequently presents with pain, redness, swelling, and warmth in the vicinity of the injury. Pus leakage and increasing discomfort are among the other symptoms that may arise from an infection of the ingrown toenail.

Appropriate care and therapy can help reduce the symptoms and avoid consequences. It may involve lifestyle changes, at-home remedies, or, in extreme circumstances, medical intervention. It's critical to seek medical assistance, particularly if the ingrown toenail is recurrent, connected to an infection, or if the feet are affected by underlying medical disorders.

Ingrown toenail risk can be decreased by taking preventive steps including wearing shoes that fit properly, taking good care of your feet, and trimming your nails correctly. Treating ingrown toenails and advancing general foot health require early detection and effective care.

CHAPTER ONE

What Ingrown Toenail Means

A frequent foot condition called ingrown toenails, sometimes called onychocryptosis, occurs when a toenail's edge or corner grows into the surrounding soft tissue, usually the skin along the nail margins. This may result in the afflicted toe experiencing discomfort, redness, swelling, and inflammation. Though they can affect any toe, ingrown toenails most commonly afflict the big toe.

The illness usually appears when a toenail curls inward or pierces through the skin next to it instead of growing straight out. This could be caused by things like cutting your nails too short, wearing shoes that are too small or too tight, having a genetic tendency, injuring your toenail, or having certain illnesses that interfere with nail growth.

From slightly irritating to extremely painful, ingrown toenails can cause a varicty of symptoms. If they get infected, they may also cause increasing soreness and pus leakage.

A warm soak, suitable footwear, and at-home cures are just a few of the therapy options that might help relieve the symptoms of ingrown toenails. Medical intervention, such as expert toenail trimming, infection drainage, or, in severe situations, surgical operations to remove a section of the toenail, may be required in more severe or recurrent cases.

Wearing shoes that fit properly, avoiding footwear that is too tight, and clipping toenails straight across as opposed to rounded are all examples of preventive practices. To avoid problems and advance the general health of the foot, early detection and timely treatment are crucial.

The Toenail's Anatomy

Human toenails are hard, protective structures that cover the tips of the toes. They are also called nail plates. It is a component of the nail unit, a bigger structure made up of several different parts. An outline of the toenail's anatomy is shown below:

Plate with nails:

The nail plate is the part of the toenail that is visible and firm. It is made of keratin, a hard protein that gives the nail strength and defense.

The Nail Matrix

The tissue that lies beneath the cuticle and beneath the nail base is called the nail matrix. It is in charge of generating new nail cells, which support the nail plate's expansion and thickness.

Lunula:

The visible white patch at the base of the nail that resembles a crescent is called the lunula. It is typically easier to see on the thumbnail and represents the portion of the nail matrix that is visible. The lunula marks the site of the matrix but is not directly engaged in nail formation.

Eponychium cuticle:

To shield the nail matrix, the cuticle, a thin layer of skin, protects the base of the nail. It serves as a barrier to stop fungus and bacteria from growing within the nail matrix and infecting the skin.

Bed of nails:

Tissue under the nail plate is called the nail bed. It has blood arteries that carry nutrients to the developing nail cells and supports the nail plate structurally.

Hyponychium:

The skin region beneath the nail's free edge is known as the hyponychium. It acts as a barrier of defense, keeping dirt and microbes out of the area under the nail.

Perionychium:

The skin and soft tissues that surround the nail are part of the perionychium. It is made up of the lateral and proximal nail folds, which serve to seal the nail unit and ward off infections.

For appropriate nail hygiene and maintenance, it is imperative to comprehend the structure of the toenail. Toenail health can be improved and disorders like ingrown toenails can be avoided by wearing properly fitting shoes, following proper nail-trimming practices, and keeping up good foot hygiene.

There are several reasons and risk factors that might lead to the development of an ingrown toenail. These elements could encourage the toenail to spread into the surrounding tissue, which could result in discomfort, swelling, and even an infection. Ingrown toenail frequent causes and risk factors are as follows:

Unsuitable Nail Trimming:

The toenail may grow into the surrounding skin if it is trimmed excessively short or rounded at the edges rather than clipped straight across.

Ill-fitting or too-tight shoes:

Shoes that are excessively narrow or tight might put pressure on the toes, pushing the nail into the skin.

Toe injuries:

A toe injury or trauma, like being stubbled or having a heavy object dropped on it, might alter the toenail's growth pattern and raise the possibility of ingrown toenails.

Biological Propensity:

A genetic susceptibility to ingrown toenails may exist in some people. There could be a higher chance of getting ingrown toenails if family members have a history of them.

Unusual Nail Form:

An increased risk of ingrown toenails can be associated with specific nail forms, such as curved or involuted nails.

Inadequate Foot Care:

Ingrown toenails can result from poor foot hygiene, such as not cleaning or clipping the nails on a regular basis.

Sweating Too Much:

Hyperhidrosis, or excessive perspiration on the foot, can weaken the skin around toenails, increasing the risk of nail penetration.

Basis Conditions:

An increased risk of ingrown toenails can result from conditions that interfere with nail growth, such as fungal infections or specific nail abnormalities.

Unsuitable Footwear:

High heels or shoes with a small toe box can squeeze the toes and increase the risk of ingrown toenails.

Gender and Age:

Ingrown toenails are more common in adolescents and young adults, and they affect more men than women.

Diseases of the System:

Peripheral artery disease and diabetes, for example, are examples of systemic disorders that can impair circulation and raise the risk of foot issues, including ingrown toenails.

Changes in Hormones:

Changes in hormones brought on by menopause, adolescence, or pregnancy might affect nail growth and make ingrown toenails more likely.

By being aware of these causes and risk factors, people can lower their chance of having ingrown toenails by taking preventative actions and maintaining excellent foot hygiene. For the correct diagnosis and treatment, it's critical to seek medical assistance if ingrown toenails become severe, recurrent, or infected.

Symptoms and Indications

Ingrown toenails can be painful and present with a range of symptoms, frequently affecting the big toe. The following are typical indications and symptoms of ingrown toenails:

Suffering and Sensitivity:

An ingrown toenail often causes pain along the side of the nail. The afflicted region could feel sensitive to pressure.

Swelling and Redness:

Because of irritation and inflammation, the skin surrounding the ingrown toenail may become red and swollen.

Warmth:

Warmth that is increased around the ingrown toenail indicates inflammation, particularly in cases where an infection is present.

Pus Drainage:

When an ingrown toenail is infected, pus or drainage may come out of it. Tenderness and pain may worsen in tandem with this.

Trouble Putting on Shoes:

It may be difficult to wear shoes comfortably due to the pain and swelling caused by an ingrown toenail.

Skin (Granulation Tissue) Overgrowth:

Granulation tissue may eventually form around the ingrown toenail as a result of the body's overproduction of tissue in response to the irritation.

Hemorrhaging:

If the skin around the ingrown toenail is damaged, there may be some bleeding.

Nail Shape Changes:

The damaged nail may change in shape as a result of the ingrown toenail, especially if there is nail penetration into the epidermis.

Suffering under Pressure:

Walking or wearing tight shoes can put pressure on the ingrown toenail, which can make pain and discomfort worse.

Bad Smell:

An unpleasant smell connected to the ingrown toenail may be present in cases of infection.

It's crucial to remember that if the ingrown toenail gets infected, symptoms could get worse and there might be other indications of the infection, such fever or spreading redness. People with persistent ingrown toenails, evidence of infection, or excruciating pain should visit a doctor. To treat the ingrown toenail, offer relief, and avoid complications, medical intervention can be required in certain situations.

CHAPTER TWO

Identification

An ingrown toenail is usually diagnosed by examining the affected toe physically and talking about the patient's symptoms and medical background. The following diagnostic techniques can be used by medical professionals, such as podiatrists or general practitioners, to evaluate and identify ingrown toenails:

Clinical Assessment:

The medical professional will visually examine the afflicted toe, searching for indications of inflammation, redness, soreness, and any obvious evidence of the toenail expanding into the surrounding tissue.

Health Background:

A thorough medical history will be taken, encompassing details regarding the development of symptoms, any injuries or trigger events, and any prior instances of ingrown toenails.

Evaluation of Symptoms:

The degree and impact on everyday activities of the individual's stated symptoms, including pain, soreness, and trouble putting on shoes, will be evaluated.

Physical Deception:

To evaluate the damaged toenail's mobility, look for infection symptoms, and gauge the amount of ingrowth, the healthcare professional may gently manipulate the affected nail.

Evaluation of the Adjacent Tissues:

We will look for indications of infection, inflammation, or granulation tissue on the skin surrounding the ingrown toenail.

Imaging studies, if appropriate:

For the most part, identifying ingrown toenails does not require imaging studies like X-rays. However, imaging might be advised if complications are suspected or if there are worries about the involvement of the underlying bone.

Evaluation of Nail Form:

To find any contributing factors, the healthcare provider may examine the toenail's shape and ask about nail-trimming practices.

Assessment of Root Causes:

Further evaluations may be carried out to treat the underlying cause if ingrown toenails are recurrent or linked to an underlying illness (such as systemic diseases or nail problems).

People should be transparent in their communication with their healthcare provider, sharing information about their symptoms and any attempts at self-care at home. This data facilitates precise diagnosis and directs the creation of a suitable treatment strategy.

Seeking professional medical attention is essential in cases of severe discomfort, infection, or recurring ingrown toenails. In order to address the ingrown toenail and provide relief, healthcare experts may recommend a variety of treatments, including as conservative methods, small operations (such partial nail removal), or, in rare circumstances, surgical interventions. Prompt diagnosis and prompt management can aid in averting problems and expediting recuperation.

Options for Treatment

The severity of the problem and the presence of any related infection determine how to treat an ingrown toenail. The following are some methods of treating ingrown toenails:

Warm Baths:

One way to help lessen discomfort and reduce inflammation in the affected foot is to soak it in warm water. This is usually done a few times a day for fifteen to twenty minutes.

Suitable Nail Trimming:

Preventing more ingrowth can be achieved by making sure to trim toenails straight across, without rounding the edges. Steer clear of shoes that are too small or poorly fitting.

Dental floss or cotton wedge:

To encourage healthy growth, you can raise the ingrown toenail away from the epidermis by placing a little piece of cotton or dental floss under it. After the foot has been soaked, this can be done.

Topical Antibiotics:

Preventing infection can be achieved by using antibiotic ointments purchased over-the-counter to the affected area. It is imperative to maintain the space tidy.

Medication for Pain:

Acetaminophen and ibuprofen, two over-the-counter pain medications, can help lessen discomfort and inflammation.

Steer Clear of Tight Shoes:

It is possible to avoid putting further strain on the toenail by donning shoes that fit comfortably and have enough room for the toes.

Professional Trimming of Nails:

Podiatrists among other healthcare professionals are capable of cutting or extracting the ingrown toenail. This is frequently carried out in a controlled setting with sterile tools.

Braces or splints for nails:

To allow for healthy growth, the medical professional may occasionally employ braces or splints to raise an ingrown toenail away from the epidermis.

Removal of Some Nails (Matrixectomy):

A doctor might advise partial nail extraction if the ingrown toenails are severe or recurrent. This entails cutting off a section of the ingrown edge of the toenail. There are a few different ways to accomplish this, such as chemical matrixectomy or surgical excision.

Antibiotic-Related Drugs:

The medical professional may recommend oral antibiotics to treat any infection that may be present.

Surgical Procedure:

Surgical techniques like complete nail avulsion or partial nail avulsion combined with matrixectomy may be taken into consideration for severe or persistent instances. Local anesthetic is usually used during these procedures.

People who have ingrown toenails should consult a doctor, especially if there are indications of an infection or if self-care remedies aren't working. Complications may arise if severe or infected ingrown toenails are attempted to be treated on oneself at home.

Wearing shoes that fit properly, taking care of your nails, and addressing contributing factors are among preventive steps that can help lower your chance of ingrown toenails. To avoid complications, people with diabetes or circulatory problems should get medical assistance for ingrown toenails as soon as possible.

Taking proper care of your feet and changing your lifestyle can help prevent ingrown toenails by lowering your risk of toenail-related problems. The following are some methods to avoid having ingrown toenails:

Suitable Nail Trimming:

Cut toenails squarely, without rounding off corners. Trim the nails not too short, but in the shape of the toe. A good nail clipper should be used, and the nails should not be torn or pulled.

Foot Care:

Maintain dry, clean feet. After taking a bath, wash your feet frequently and make sure to completely dry them, especially in between your toes.

Appropriate Size for Shoes:

Put on shoes that fit properly and have adequate space for your toes. Steer clear of shoes with a pointed toe box, excessive tightness, or narrowness.

Keep Your Hosiery Tight:

Opt for loose-fitting socks or undergarments, as this may lead to pressure points on the toes and escalate the possibility of ingrown toenails.

Footwear that protects:

Wherever there is a chance of toe injuries, including during sports or strenuous physical activity, wear protective footwear.

Frequent examinations of the feet:

Regularly check the feet for anomalies such as redness, edema, or ingrown toenails. Prompt intervention is made possible by early detection.

The Right Method for Cutting Nails:

Instead of cutting toenails in a curved or rounded shape, cut them straight across. Steer clear of cutting into the toenail corners.

Steer clear of toe trauma:

To prevent ingrown toenails, take care not to injure or traumatize your toes. When the toes are in danger, make sure they are protected.

Foot Exercises:

To keep your feet flexible and avoid abnormalities that could lead to ingrown toenails, do foot exercises.

Products for Healthy Nail Care:

Use nail care products that are mild and non-irritating. Steer clear of cutting cuticles too quickly or utilizing sharp things close to the toenails.

Foot Safety During Water Activities:

When engaging in water activities, including swimming or taking public showers, wear protective footwear to lower your risk of fungal infections that can damage your toenails.

Take Care of the Underlying Conditions:

Seek appropriate medical care to manage any underlying problems, such as fungal infections or systemic diseases, that may be influencing nail growth or raising the risk of ingrown toenails.

Frequent Professional Foot Care:

For professional foot care, think about scheduling routine appointments with a podiatrist or other healthcare provider, particularly if there is a history of recurring ingrown toenails.

You may lessen the chance of getting ingrown toenails and improve the general health of your feet by implementing these preventive practices into your daily foot care regimen. People who have diabetes or circulatory problems should take extra precautions when it comes to foot care and should seek medical attention as soon as they have any foot-related problems.

Difficulties

Complications may arise from ingrown toenails, particularly if they are left untreated or if an infection is present. The following are typical outcomes of ingrown toenails:

Callus (Cellulitis):

Infection is among the most frequent side effects and can happen when germs get into the space around the ingrown toenail. Pus leakage, redness, swelling, and warmth may result from this. Cellulitis could arise from the infection and cause more extensive inflammation.

Formation of Abscesses:

An abscess, or collection of pus, may arise in severe infection instances. This may exacerbate discomfort and necessitate medical assistance for drainage.

Persistent discomfort and pain:

Persistent or recurring ingrown toenails can cause long-term discomfort and agony. The constant stress and irritation could have an impact on day-to-day activities and overall well-being.

Formation of Granulation Tissue:

Granulation tissue is an extra tissue that the body produces as a reaction to long-term irritation from an ingrown toenail. This tissue may need to be managed by a professional and may exacerbate discomfort.

Bacterial infections that occur later:

Bacterial infections can become recurrent if an ingrown toenail is not treated appropriately, creating a vicious cycle of pain and irritation.

Reduced Movement:

Ingrown toenail pain can cause excruciating agony, which can make it difficult to move and walk.

Nail Shape Changes:

Persistent ingrown toenails may result in modifications to the affected toenail's shape and appearance. This could result in malformations, discolouration, or thickness.

Postponed Recovery:

Delays in healing can occur from not treating ingrown toenails as soon as possible, particularly if there are other contributing factors such impaired immune system or circulation.

Injuries:

Scarring could happen if there is a serious infection or if surgery is necessary. The look of the surrounding tissues and toenail might be impacted by scarring.

Transmission of the Infection to Neighboring **Tissues:**

In severe situations, infections brought on by ingrown toenails may spread to neighboring tissues if left untreated, which could result in more catastrophic consequences.

Rare Systemic Infections:

Severe infections that go untreated can, however rarely, result in systemic consequences like sepsis. People with compromised immune systems or other underlying medical issues are more likely to experience this.

To avoid difficulties, it's critical to treat ingrown toenails as soon as possible. It is imperative to seek expert medical assistance, particularly in cases where infection symptoms are present. To address difficulties and improve recovery, healthcare providers can administer the required interventions, such as surgical procedures, antibiotics, or drainage. To prevent major consequences, people with diabetes or circulatory problems should take extra care when taking care of their feet.

CHAPTER THREE

When to Get Medical Help

It's critical to seek medical help for an ingrown toenail, particularly if there are indications of infection or if self-care techniques are ineffective. When dealing with an ingrown toenail, it's best to get medical help right away in the following situations:

Infection Warning Signs:

Timely medical intervention is required if there are indications of infection, such as elevated redness, swelling, temperature, and pus leakage from the ingrown toenail.

Enhanced Pain and Soreness:

It's important to see a healthcare provider if the ingrown toenail pain and discomfort are significant and do not improve with at-home remedies.

Continuing Symptoms:

In case the symptoms don't go away even after trying at-home remedies like warm baths and appropriate nail cutting, a professional assessment might be required.

Recurring Ingrown Nails on Toes:

In cases where there is a history of recurrent episodes or recurrent ingrown toenails, a healthcare provider can evaluate the underlying causes and suggest suitable preventive measures.

Having Trouble Walking:

Getting medical attention is crucial for proper management if the ingrown toenail is making it difficult to walk or substantially limiting your movement.

Diabetic state:

Diabetes patients should get medical help for ingrown toenails as soon as possible since their compromised immune systems and circulation put them at higher risk of infections and consequences.

Fundamental Medical Conditions:

It is crucial to speak with a healthcare provider for thorough treatment if there are any underlying medical diseases, such as immunological disorders or peripheral artery disease, that may have an impact on the foot.

Impeded healing

A medical review is required if there are evidence of problems, delayed recovery, or poor healing.

Symptoms throughout the system:

In addition to an ingrown toenail, systemic symptoms like fever, chills, or malaise could point to a more serious infection that has to be treated by a doctor.

Possibly Abscess:

In the event that an abscess (a collection of pus) is suspected around the ingrown toenail, drainage may be necessary as part of medical care.

Aggressive self-treatment should be avoided, particularly if the ingrown toenail is causing a great deal of discomfort or there are indications of infection. Podiatrists are among the healthcare professionals who can provide suitable interventions to treat ingrown toenails and avoid complications. These interventions may include professional nail trimming, drainage, or, in extreme circumstances, surgical procedures. Effective management and limiting the worsening of symptoms depend on early intervention.

Ingrown toenail management and prevention can be achieved by implementing specific lifestyle changes. Here are some practices and lifestyle adjustments to think about:

Suitable Nail Trimming:

Keep your toenails neat and square, without any rounded corners. Don't cut them too short; instead, shape them to resemble a toe. To avoid jagged edges, use the right nail clippers.

Foot Care:

Maintain dry, clean feet. After taking a bath, wash them frequently and make sure they are completely dry, especially in between the toes.

Fitting Footwear:

Put on shoes that fit properly and allow space for your toes. In order to avoid putting pressure on the toenails, choose shoes with a wide toe box. Steer clear of narrow or tight shoes.

Footwear that protects:

When playing sports or engaging in strenuous physical activity, or anywhere else where your toes could be injured, wear protective footwear.

Frequent examinations of the feet:

Regularly examine your feet for any irregularities, such as redness, swelling, or ingrown toenails. Prompt intervention is made possible by early detection.

Foot Exercises:

Engage in activities that enhance the strength and flexibility of your feet. By doing this, abnormalities that could lead to ingrown toenails can be avoided.

Sustain a Healthy Weight:

One factor that might cause pressure on the toes is excess body weight. The likelihood of ingrown toenails can be decreased by maintaining a healthy weight.

Precautionary Steps for Activities in Water:

When engaging in water activities, including swimming or taking public showers, wear protective footwear to lower your risk of fungal infections that can damage your toenails.

Frequent Professional Foot Care:

For professional foot care, think about scheduling routine appointments with a podiatrist or other healthcare provider, particularly if there is a history of recurring ingrown toenails.

Select the Correct Socks:

Avoid wearing too-tight socks or other hosiery since this can put pressure on the toes and raise the possibility of ingrown toenails.

Steer clear of toe trauma:

Take care to prevent toe trauma or injury. When your toes could be in danger, take precautions to keep them safe.

Products for Healthy Nail Care:

Use nail care products that are mild and non-irritating. Steer clear of cutting cuticles too quickly or utilizing sharp things close to the toenails.

Take Care of the Underlying Conditions:

Seek appropriate medical care to manage any underlying problems, such as fungal infections or systemic diseases, that may be influencing nail growth or raising the risk of ingrown toenails.

When regularly followed, these lifestyle changes can help prevent ingrown toenails and improve the general health of your feet. See a medical expert for advice and the best course of action if you frequently or severely suffer from ingrown toenails.

CONCLUSION

In conclusion, ingrown toenails can cause pain and discomfort, but they can also be managed and avoided with the right care. The secret is to acquire healthy foot care habits, modify one's lifestyle, and seek prompt medical help when necessary.

Preventing ingrown toenails primarily involves wearing appropriate footwear, keeping your feet clean, and cutting your nails properly. Early detection and treatment of the illness can help prevent it from getting worse. Regular foot exams can assist.

In cases when there are indications of infection, ongoing pain, or difficulty walking, it's critical to get help. Podiatrists are among the healthcare professionals who can give a range of therapies, including surgical operations, professional nail trimming, and drainage, to treat ingrown toenails and avoid problems.

A healthy weight, toe protection, and workouts that increase foot flexibility are some of the lifestyle modifications that help avoid ingrown toenails generally. Maintaining foot health requires regular professional visits, consistent foot care, and treatment of underlying issues.

Through proactive and aware foot care habits, people can lessen discomfort, lower their chance of ingrown toenails, and improve their feet's general health. Consulting with medical professionals guarantees proper diagnosis and treatment for the best possible results if ingrown toenails are persistent or cause worries.

THE END